Complete Walkthrough On

VARDENAFIL

Steven Kane

VARDENAFIL GUIDE

Vardenafil, also known as Levitra, is a prescription medication that is used to treat male erectile dysfunction. There are benefits and drawbacks to taking Vardenafil.

When a man can't get or keep an erection, he has erectile dysfunction. It normally happens in light of the fact that the conduits that convey the blood to the penis are excessively tight.

Vardenafil increments blood stream to the penis.

Levitra has a similar effect to Viagra, which lasts between 2 and 4 hours, while Viagra lasts between 2 and 4 hours.

How can it function?

A man can get and keep an erection with Vardenafil.

During a penile erection, the penis loads up with blood.

The blood vessels that take blood away from the penis contract while the blood vessels that supply the penis with blood expand, or dilate. The corpus cavernosa, or two large penis chambers, are filled with blood.

An erection occurs as the blood builds up in the penis.

Vardenafil is a member of the phosphodiesterase type-5 (PDE5) inhibitors class of drugs. PDE5 is stopped from constricting the arteries by a PDE5 inhibitor.

Vardenafil increases blood flow when a man is sexually stimulated by relaxing the arteries.

During arousal, the active ingredient affects the penis's reaction chain.

Nitric oxide is released into a man's penis when he is sexually stimulated, triggering a series of reactions.

Cyclic guanosine monophosphate, or cGMP, is produced as a result by an enzyme known as guanylate cyclase.

The blood vessels that carry blood to and from the penis are regulated by cGMP through contraction and dilation, or expansion. The vessels that remove blood from the penis contract while the vessels that supply the penis expand as a result of the chemical reaction.

Phosphodiesterase-5 (PDE5), another chemical separates or annihilates cGMP.

The blood vessels return to their normal size when cGMP is destroyed, effectively ending the erection. Vardenafil prevents cGMP destruction by PDE5. It prolongs the lifespan of cGMP in this manner. Therefore, it draws out an erection.

Vardenafil comes in tablets with doses of 2.5 milligrams (mg), 5 mg, 10 mg, and 20 mg. Typically, the first dose is 10 mg.

A dose of vardenafil of 10 milligrams is roughly equivalent to 50 milligrams of Viagra or sildenafil. This is due to the fact that vardenafil and sildenafil have distinct chemical compositions.

Vardenafil is required 25 to an hour prior to sex. The result can last up to five hours. Every 24 hours, only one tablet can be taken.

Before swallowing orodispersible tablets, they must be allowed to dissolve on the tongue. They shouldn't be taken with drinks of any kind.

Since the drug won't work unless the man is sexually stimulated, foreplay is usually required.

Vardenafil can be taken with or without food, but you shouldn't drink alcohol because it makes it harder to get an erection. Liquor can likewise expand the gamble of unfriendly impacts.

Alerts

Likewise with all drugs, unfavorable impacts and cooperations can happen while utilizing vardenafil.

Men will experience headaches one in ten times.

Other symptoms that are common include:

A stuffy or swollen nose; stomach pain; dizziness; flushing; these symptoms typically go away within a few hours.

Other signs that could be dangerous include:

Ringing in the ears, sudden loss of hearing, irregular heartbeat, swelling of the ankles, hands, or feet, difficulty breathing, or chest pain. If any of these things happen, the patient should stop taking vardenafil.

An allergic reaction is uncommon. This can prompt hives, trouble breathing, and expanding of the face, tongue, and throat. It has the potential to shock and kill. It should be treated as a medical emergency if these symptoms appear.

Priapism is a very uncommon side effect that occurs when an erection lasts longer than four hours. The penis may be harmed by this. Assuming that an erection endures too lengthy, the individual ought to look for clinical consideration.

Visual disturbances

A drop in eye blood pressure can cause visual disturbances. The individual might notice that things have a blue tint to them, and they might have trouble telling the difference between green and blue.

Rarely, one or both eyes may experience a sudden loss of vision. This can demonstrate a heart condition, a current eye issue, elevated cholesterol, diabetes, or hypertension.

Assuming that any unexpected loss of vision happens, the individual ought to quit taking the medicine and look for clinical assistance right away.

Patients who suffer from diabetes, high cholesterol, or heart or coronary artery disease are more likely to experience vision issues. If a person smokes or is over 50, they are more likely to develop vision problems.

Using Vardenafil in conjunction with other medications can result in serious side effects.

Among the possible responses are:

- a possibly hazardous drop in pulse, or hypotension
- wooziness
- blacking out

There is likewise a gamble of stroke and coronary episode.

Vardenafil should not be taken by men who are taking nitrate medications for chest pain or heart problems, such as riociguat (Adempas).

It ought not to be utilized with the sporting medications, amyl nitrate and butyl nitrate, otherwise called poppers.

Other drugs that could interact with one another include, but are not limited to:

Grapefruit juice contains a chemical that increases the likelihood of adverse effects, so it should not be consumed while taking vardenafil. Other medications for erectile dysfunction, prostate problems, blood pressure, or heart rhythm disorders, and antibiotics and antifungal medications are also prohibited.

Before taking Vardenafil, patients should discuss all of their medical conditions with their doctor, as well as any other medications or supplements they take.

This is particularly crucial if they have:

a heart condition such as arrhythmia, heart failure, or angina; a family history of a rare heart condition known as long QT syndrome; hearing problems; hemophilia or some kind of bleeding problem; hypotension (low blood pressure) or hypertension (high blood pressure); liver or kidney problems;

multiple myeloma, leukemia, sickle cell anemia, or some other kind of blood cell problem; non-arteritic anterior ischemic optic neuropathy (NAION

Levitra can be bought online, but users should think about the aforementioned points and talk to their doctor first.

Is CBD effective against erectile dysfunction?

The compound known as cannabidiol (CBD) is derived from the cannabis plant. It may help alleviate anxiety, stress, and depression symptoms, according to some evidence. These circumstances might make individuals more inclined to creating erectile brokenness (ED).

CBD items are accessible in numerous skin structures, like creams, salves, and greases that people can apply to their penis. However, a person with ED might want to talk to a doctor about the condition's treatment and the safety of CBD.

The use of CBD is covered in greater detail in this article. It takes a gander at the advantages and dangers of CBD for ED, as well as different medicines that might ease erectile issues.

Is CBD effective against erectile dysfunction?

Getty Images, a 2018 study by Trusted Source suggests that CBD may alleviate symptoms of the following conditions:

- persistent agony
- rest problems
- headache
- joint inflammation

There is no proof straightforwardly supporting the utilization of CBD to treat ED. Notwithstanding, CBD might furnish some help in individuals with specific medical issues that might be risk factors for ED.

Studies on CBD for erectile dysfunction

The effectiveness of cannabinoids is being evaluated by researchers to see if they can alleviate symptoms in people with multiple sclerosis. This is a drawn out condition that causes dizziness, vision issues, quakes, and exhaustion, among different side effects. There is trust that if cannabinoids can assist with treating MS side effects, these patients can stay away from normal MS meds that lead to ED.

ED may occur in MS patients, but this may be a side effect of their medication.

According to a Trusted Source study from 2021, men with anxiety disorders are more likely to experience ED.

Another investigation discovered that CBD might have energizer, antipsychotic, and antiepileptic impacts. This demonstrates that it may be a treatment option for anxiety-related symptoms, which could be beneficial to those with anxiety-induced ED.

Chronic stress, personality disorders, and difficulties in relationships are also thought by some researchers to be risk factors for ED. According to a 2019 study, individuals with post-traumatic stress disorder (PTSD) may benefit from taking CBD orally to lessen the severity of their symptoms. In any case, it might furnish more noteworthy advantages in mix with mental meetings.

Dive more deeply into different enhancements for ED.

How it works: CBD may be able to reduce pain.

The endocannabinoid system, which controls various functions like appetite, emotional behavior, pain sensation, and memory, is found in the human body.

Endocannabinoids are neurotransmitters produced by the body that bind to cannabinoid receptors in the nervous system.

Studies show that CBD might influence endocannabinoid receptor movement. People who suffer from chronic pain may benefit from this reduction in inflammation.

Instructions to involve CBD for erectile brokenness

CBD items come in various structures. Tropical oils and lubricants, for example, are intended for topical application and claim to increase circulation. There are likewise chewy candies, biting gums, and creams.

The following are some of the businesses that sell CBD products:

Charlotte's Web Joy Organics Lazarus Naturals cbdMD

Before making a purchase, make sure to check the price, list of ingredients, and dosage.

It very well might be really smart to check the cost, fixing rundown, and portion prior to focusing on a buy.

CBD is likewise accessible in three kinds that contain various measures of cannabinoids:

Full range: This incorporates every one of the parts that come from the marijuana plant. Additionally, it has less than 0.3 percent THC.

Spectrum wide: This may contain a small amount of THC, but it contains the majority of the plant's compounds.

Isolate: This just holds back CBD. Items don't contain THC or other cannabinoids.

Benefits CBD may offer additional advantages. In rats with diabetes, one study suggests that CBD may help reduce nerve inflammation.

According to a 2019 study conducted by Trusted Source on the effects of CBD on sleep and anxiety, a dose of 300–600 milligrams (mg) may assist in lowering cortisol levels. This demonstrates that CBD might make a soothing difference, as higher dosages might help people with epilepsy, a sleeping disorder, or tension.

However, it's possible that the outcomes weren't accurate. According to the researchers, the majority of participants were also receiving psychiatric treatment, which may have affected the outcomes.

According to Research, CBD can also help people who are quitting smoking to avoid cravings.

Chances

The World Wellbeing Association (WHO) expresses that CBD is protected, and most secondary effects happen when individuals use it in blend with different medications. In point of fact, CBD is being promoted as a medical product in some nations.

The Food and Medication Organization (FDA) specifies the potential aftereffects that CBD can cause. These include:

- liver injury
- richness issues in guys
- looseness of the bowels
- touchiness

Likewise, it could be best for individuals to look for clinical counsel prior to purchasing a CBD item, as not all have gone through the FDA's endorsement interaction.

According to Trusted Source, the FDA has only approved one product derived from cannabis and three synthetic products related to cannabis. You can get these with a prescription.

Treatments for erectile dysfunction

The trusted source from the National Institute of Diabetes and Digestive and Kidney Diseases (NIDDK) talks about self-care advice, medications, and devices that could help treat ED.

Tips for self-care Individuals who struggle with erectile dysfunction might want to consider the following:

Medications Doctors may prescribe medications that increase blood flow in the penis during stimulation. These include quitting smoking, if applicable, limiting alcohol consumption, engaging in regular physical activity, and increasing consumption of fruits and vegetables. Tadalafil, sildenafil, and vardenafil are examples of these.

People who are taking nitrates and have heart problems might not find these safe. A sudden drop in blood pressure may result from these drugs interfering with ED treatments.

Pumps that stimulate blood flow to the penis to induce an erection are known as vacuum pumps. A pump may be suggested by medical professionals for up to 30 minutes; from that point forward, an individual might be bound to foster skin disturbance.

Medical procedure

A few people might go through a medical procedure where an urologist embeds a gadget that assists them with keeping an erection. A person may be able to use the device after four to six weeks, and this takes place in a hospital.

In other instances, the procedure might involve reconstructing an artery, which might be best for people under the age of 30. In order to remove blockages that may be restricting blood flow to the penis, doctors repair the arteries.

In conclusion, there are no studies that demonstrate that CBD products are safe and effective in treating erectile dysfunction (ED). Notwithstanding, CBD might assist with freeing side effects from gloom, nervousness, or stress that can improve an individual's probability of creating erectile issues.

Different kinds of CBD products are available from businesses like Lazarus Naturals, Joy Organics, and Charlotte's Web. Because the FDA does not regulate all CBD products, these might not be safe for everyone.

People with ED may be able to achieve and maintain an erection with the assistance of medications, surgery, and home remedies.

Roman versus Hims: Hims and Roman are telehealth businesses that offer prescription and nonprescription treatments for erectile dysfunction (ED), hair loss, and premature ejaculation (PE). Their products, services, prices, and customer reviews are all listed below.

Both erectile dysfunction (ED) and hair loss are common health problems, with ED affecting most Trusted Source men over the age of 40 and hair loss caused by hormonal changes affecting up to 50% of Trusted Source men.

Emotional distress can result from both ED and hair loss, but both conditions can be treated with a variety of prescription medications.

These treatments from Hims and Roman can be ordered online.

This article provides responses to some frequently asked questions and discusses both brands, their products, and ordering procedures.

Please be aware that the author of this article has not used these items. All data introduced is absolutely research-based and was right at the hour of distribution.

Hims

Hims has its headquarters in San Francisco and began operations in 2017. Treatments for ED, hair loss, and PE are just a few of the conditions for which the company offers both prescription and nonprescription options. Hims is a sister company to Hers, which sells products for female health.

Hims also sells medications for mental health conditions and skin care products, such as those for wrinkles, acne, and aging support. In addition, Hims offers individual and group therapy sessions as well as psychiatric assessments.

Since Hims is a subscription service, patients typically receive their treatment once every three months or every other month.

Consider the service's advantages and disadvantages before placing an order with Hims.

Pros and cons of Him: There are many products for male health.

Both brand-name and generic medications are available.

Hims states its interviews are free.

The organization guarantees its delivery is free.

For some medications, subscribers can choose a subscription service.

Cons

Some reviewers had difficulty communicating with the customer service representatives.

Prices for all of the products on the website are unclear.

Some of its medications cost significantly more than its competitors.

It may take longer for orders to arrive than orders from competitors.

Not all going bald items are supported by the Food and Medication Organization (FDA).

On the BBB, the average customer review rating is low for it.

Roman, a New York-based business, also opened in 2017. Prescription and nonprescription treatments for ED, PE, and hair loss are offered by the business.

Additionally, Roman offers treatments for eczema and excessive sweating, two skin conditions. Additionally, it offers products for prostate health, stress relief, and testosterone support, as well as multivitamins and other daily health supplements.

Roman is a subscription business as well. Individuals will accept their treatment on request, month to month, or at regular intervals.

The benefits and drawbacks listed below should be taken into consideration before placing an order with Roman.

Roman benefits and drawbacks

- It treats a wide range of health issues.
- It provides generic and brand-name medications.
- In some cases, its medicines cost less than those of its rivals.
- The business claims to offer fast, free shipping.
- Its membership administration might be advantageous.
- It provides ongoing support and a complimentary initial consultation.

Cons

A few clients found dropping the membership troublesome.

Customers complain that they can't pick their doctors easily.

According to reviews, the business made unauthorized charges.

On the BBB, the average customer review rating is low for it.

Online customer feedback and the reputation of the brand are mixed for Hims and Roman. Study the standing of the two brands underneath.

Hims

Hims has a BBB-accredited page. The business received an A+ rating from the BBB at the time of publication. However, the average rating of customer reviews was 1.08 out of 5.

When issues arise with orders, praise for Hims is expressed in terms of their prompt responses. However, issues with canceling subscriptions, canceled appointments, and slow responses from doctors are mentioned in both neutral and negative reviews.

Commentators on Trustpilot provided Hims with a typical rating of 3.9 out of 5 stars. 69% of the 1,344 reviews here are five stars.

Customers praise doctors for providing prompt, courteous service and effective medication. Critical reviews, on the other hand, complain that customers were being charged after canceling orders and that shipping times were longer than advertised.

The ease of use and knowledgeable doctors of the service are frequently mentioned in positive reviews. According to negative feedback, it is difficult to cancel subscriptions and communication with customer service representatives is poor.

The BBB has accredited Roman

Roman. The company received a B+ grade from the organization at the time of publication.

Roman, on the other hand, received an average rating of 1.75 stars from customers on the BBB website.

At the hour of distributing, there are 12 surveys on BBB. Late deliveries and medication not delivered are mentioned in critical reviews. However, the company's vitamins and ED medications are praised for their efficacy in positive reviews, and deliveries were prompt.

Despite the fact that there are only 11 reviews on this page, the average Trustpilot rating is 2.1 stars out of 5. Roman received a rating of 1 out of 5 stars from 91% of Trustpilot reviews at the time of publication.

Customers praise doctors for providing prompt, courteous service and effective medication. Critical reviews, on the other hand, complain that customers were being charged after canceling orders and that shipping times were longer than advertised.

The ease of use and knowledgeable doctors of the service are frequently mentioned in positive reviews. According to negative feedback, it is difficult to cancel subscriptions and communication with customer service representatives is poor.

The BBB has accredited Roman. The company received a B+ grade from the organization at the time of publication.

Roman, on the other hand, received an average rating of 1.75 stars from customers on the BBB website.

At the hour of distributing, there are 12 surveys on BBB. Late deliveries and medication not delivered are mentioned in critical reviews. However, the company's vitamins and ED medications are praised for their efficacy in positive reviews, and deliveries were prompt.

Despite the fact that there are only 11 reviews on this page, the average Trustpilot rating is 2.1 stars out of 5. Roman received a rating of 1 out of 5 stars from 91% of Trustpilot reviews at the time of publication.

Inconsistent delivery times, significant price hikes, and difficulties contacting customer support are all mentioned in reviews.

Treatment for erectile dysfunction Hims and Roman provide the same prescription medications for ED.

The following ED treatments are available at Hims:

Viagra

Cost range: from $139 per use, with a prescription: yes, approved by FDA: Yes, sildenafil is the brand name of this item. Its dynamic fixing is sildenafil citrate. It is a notable and exceptionally settled ED drug.

Sildenafil

Cost range: from $3 per use, with a prescription: yes, approved by FDA: yes, by increasing blood flow to the penis, this PDE5 inhibitor from a trusted source aids in the formation and maintenance of erections. It has the same active ingredient as Viagra's generic counterpart. Hims claims that because it costs 95% less than its branded counterpart, it is the company's most popular ED treatment.

Cialis

Cost range: starting at $958 per month Prescription required: yes, approved by FDA: indeed

This marked item is another PDE5 inhibitor. It is the marked form of tadalafil. Individuals can take it once every day for individuals who need progressing support with ED. It means that people don't have to plan ahead and take medication before having sex because the drug will provide support for an erection as needed.

Tadalafil

Cost range: from $82 each month

Remedy required: yes, approved by FDA: Yes, Tadalafil is Cialis' generic counterpart. It can be taken whenever needed, and Hims claims that its effects can last up to 36 hours. Although it costs less at Hims than brand-name Cialis, users will need to make sure they take it before having sex.

Stendra's cost range is: from $53 per use, with a prescription: yes, approved by FDA: Yes, Roman does not offer this particular PDE5 inhibitor. Avanafil is its active ingredient, but Hims does not provide a generic alternative.

Within 15 minutes of taking this medication, its effects may be felt.

The following ED treatment is offered for sale by Roman ED:

Viagra

Cost range: from $90 per portion

Remedy required: yes, approved by FDA: Yes, Roman offers Viagra in strengths of 25, 50, and 100 milligrams (mg). They generally cost $90 per portion.

Roman claims that its customers prefer 50 mg.

Sildenafil

Cost range: starting at $4 per dose Prescription required: yes, approved by FDA: Yes, sildenafil, the generic version of Viagra, works in the same way but costs much less per dose. It is available in doses of 25, 50, and 100 milligrams for $4, $6, and $10, respectively.

For PE, Hims also recommends sildenafil.

Cialis

Cost range: starting at $20 per dose Prescription required: yes, approved by FDA: Yes, Cialis comes in strengths of 5, 10, and 20 milligrams from Roman. Doses of 5 mg cost $20 per pill, while doses of 10 mg and 20 mg cost $80.

Tadalafil's cost range is: from $11

Remedy required: yes, approved by FDA: indeed

With a similar dynamic fixing as Cialis, tadalafil is a more reasonable, nonexclusive as-and-when choice. It costs between $11 and $44 and comes in strengths of 5, 10, and 20 mg.

Cost of Generic

Cialis per Day: from $8 requires a prescription: yes, approved by FDA: indeed

Individuals ought to take this tadalafil drug day to day. The two dosages, 2.5 and 5 mg, cost $8 per pill.

Going bald treatment

Hims and Roman sell solution and nonprescription medicines for balding.

Hims's prescription hair loss treatments include the following:

Oral finasteride

Cost range: starting at $22 a month Prescription required: yes, approved by FDA: indeed

This pill might assist with forestalling new going bald by preventing testosterone from switching over completely to dihydrotestosterone (DHT). More significant levels of DHT can forestall new hair development.

Price range for Minoxidil Foam or Solution: starting at $15 per month Prescription required: yes, approved by FDA: Yes, another treatment that may help prevent hair loss is Minoxidil (Rogaine). This prescription urges hair to stay in the developing stage and keeps hair from dropping out of the follicles.

Hims provides minoxidil in the form of a foam or solution. Hims claims that the foam can show results in three to six months, and that it may be easier to apply. Nonetheless, it is more costly at $20-30 for every jug.

Hims claims that the crown of the head is the most suitable area for the minoxidil solution. It costs $15 per bottle.

Spray containing finasteride and minoxidil no listed price Prescription required: yes, approved by FDA: no

This shower consolidates finasteride and minoxidil to give the advantages of both FDA-supported meds. Nonetheless, this shower isn't FDA-endorsed.

Directions encourage individuals to shower this onto their hair one time per day and they might get results inside 3-6 months.

Price range for Thick Fix Thickening Shampoo and Conditioner: from $19 per bottle

Solution required: without FDA approval: Saw palmetto, which has been implicated in research as a potential natural remedy for hair loss, is the ingredient in no Hims' Thickening Shampoo. However, additional research is required, and this shampoo may only appear to thicken hair.

Eah bottle of the Thickening Conditioner costs $22. Niacinamide is used to hydrate the hair. It gives your hair a softer, fuller appearance.

Roman balding

Roman has the accompanying balding medicines accessible:

Oral finasteride

Cost range: $20 per month requires a prescription: yes, approved by FDA: Yes, Propecia is sold under the generic name Finasteride. It can assist with easing back balding.

Effective minoxidil

Cost range: $16 per month requires a prescription: yes, approved by FDA: Yes, Roman recommends applying this topical treatment to the head's crown. It might aid in hair regrow.

Oral minoxidil

Cost range: $30 per month

Remedy required: yes, approved by FDA: no, oral minoxidil is considered an off-label use of minoxidil despite its FDA approval. This indicates that the FDA has not approved its use for hair loss in this form.

According to Roman, it has the same components as topical minoxidil but may cause distinct side effects like low blood pressure and leg swelling.

Price range for finasteride and minoxidil: $35 every month

Solution required: yes, approved by FDA: yes, oral finasteride and topical minoxidil are included in this package. This furnishes an individual with the advantages of the two medications: finasteride can slow balding, while minoxidil can assist with regrowing hair.

Treatment for premature ejaculation Hims and Roman both offer wipes and sprays as treatments for PE.

Hims provides both prescription and nonprescription PE treatment at Hims.

Cost of Climax Delay Spray: $31 per bottle Need a prescription: without FDA approval: No Climax Delay Spray is a desensitizing spray that people can use to delay ejaculation without a prescription. Lidocaine, a local anesthetic, is used.

Sertraline, an antidepressant, is also available from Hims to treat PE.

Cost of Climax Delay Wipes: $19 per wipe Need a prescription: without FDA approval: Similar to the spray, no Climax Delay Wipes work. Benzocaine, a common local anesthetic used to alleviate pain and delay orgasm, is present in each wipe. They might be a less muddled method for utilizing effective PE items.

Antidepressants cost from: $24 per month

Requires a prescription: yes, approved by FDA: not so much for PE

Hims offers two antidepressants as off-mark medicines for PE. Sertraline and paroxetine are two examples.

Antidepressants are known to reduce charisma, which might assist an individual with postponing discharge. However, ED can also result from them.

Hims offers these antidepressants for use in the treatment of PE off-label despite the fact that they are approved by the FDA to treat anxiety and depression.

Roman untimely discharge

Roman's solution and nonprescription medicines for PE include:

Roman Swipes are priced at: starting at $22 a month Prescription required: without FDA approval: The desensitizing product known as no Roman Swipes can be applied to the penis to help delay ejaculation. 4% benzocaine is used.

Products sprayed with benzocaine from Trusted Source have not been approved by the FDA. There are eight single-use wipes in each box.

Price range for Sertraline: from $0.80 per portion

Remedy required: without FDA approval: Roman does not provide an antidepressant for PE: sertraline. This medication must be taken every day, and people should be aware that it can have serious side effects.

How to Order

While nonprescription items can be ordered directly from the Hims and Roman websites, prescription medications require additional steps.

Seeking Hims solution medicines

To arrange a solution treatment, individuals should make a record with Hims and examine their side effects with an authorized medical services proficient. This interview happens on the web.

A prescription can be written if the medical professional determines that the medication is appropriate. After that, Hims discreetly ships the medication to the individual. The package is delivered in two to five business days and is sent for free.

Hims provides ongoing care and free consultations. However, these services are not covered by insurance companies.

Obtaining Roman prescription treatments

To order Roman prescription treatments, a person must upload a picture of their ID and complete an online questionnaire about their symptoms and medical history.

A healthcare professional examines this questionnaire to determine the best course of action and, if necessary, issues a prescription.

Roman provides follow-up appointments without charge. These appointments and treatments are not covered by insurance.

The business provides discrete, cost-free shipping. Roman writes that customers will receive their packages between two and four days after placing their orders. However, all orders are eligible for free two-day shipping.

How do Hims and Roman look at?

The products and services offered by Hims and Roman are comparable. We present a more in-depth comparison of the two businesses below.

While Hims lists some prices but not others, Price Roman has a pricing page for all of its products on its website.

The table beneath shows how Hims and Roman look at on costs for medicines for ED, going bald, and PE.

As of April 2023, the prices are correct.

Hims offers Roman Viagra for $139 per dose or $90 per dose; Sildenafil for $3 per dose or $4 per dose; oral finasteride for $22 per month or $20 per month; topical minoxidil for $15 per month or $16 per month; and PE wipes for $19 per wipe or $22 per month. Products and conditions

Beauty tips: Acne creams, support for aging, and basic skin care products are all included in this.

Allergies: Hims treats hay fever, itchy eyes, sinus congestion, and seasonal allergies.

Infections: Hims offers treatments for a variety of conditions, including ringworm, jock itch, athlete's foot, yeast infections, and urinary tract infections (UTIs).

Depression and anxiousness: Different energizer meds are accessible following a conference.

Treatment and care groups: Hims provides online, anonymous support groups and online counseling with licensed therapists for $99 per session.

Roman provides the following additional goods:

Mouth blisters and genital herpes: Valacyclovir, an antiviral, is provided by Roman.

Supplements taken daily: Roman can give a men's multivitamin and day to day supplements for heart wellbeing, testosterone support, stress help, and prostate wellbeing.

Allergies: Different enemy of sensitivity meds are accessible beginning at $19 each month.

Eczema: On a quarterly basis, prescription tramcinolone cream is available.

A lot of sweating: Hyperhidrosis, or excessive sweating, can be treated with a prescription-only topical product.

Emotional well-being: Depression, anxiety, and seasonal affective disorder (SAD) can all be treated with Roman.

Weight control: Roman prescribes Plenity, which it claims is the only weight management tool approved by the FDA made from natural building blocks.

Consultations

Both businesses provide complimentary initial and ongoing appointments.

Insurance, delivery, and subscriptions

Both businesses provide subscriptions on a monthly or quarterly basis. Roman also lets people buy certain things when they want to.

Hims and Roman provide discreet, free delivery.

Both services do not take insurance.

Concerns regarding safety Hims and Roman offer safety information for all products. An overview of some of the potential side effects of taking Hims or Roman medication is provided below.

Results of ED drug

A few normal results of ED drug include:

The National Institute of Diabetes and Digestive and Kidney Diseases (NIDDK) Trusted Source also advises seeking medical attention if a person's ED medication causes a prolonged erection or if they experience vision or hearing loss. Other symptoms include sensitivity to light and headaches.

Side effects of medications for hair loss Both Hims and Roman offer finasteride for hair loss. Finasteride has a number of common side effects, including Trusted Source:

ED decrease in ejaculate volume increase in the risk of high-grade prostate cancer if a person takes any other medication, they should tell the doctor or nurse during their appointment. There are some drugs that can cause problems with other medicines that could make things worse or even kill you.

For instance, people who take nitrates and PDE5 inhibitors to treat erectile dysfunction (ED) are more likely to develop potentially fatal low blood pressure, according to Trusted Source

Alternatives

The following telehealth companies can be considered alternatives to Hims and Roman:

Keeps: Keeps offers a variety of thickening shampoos, conditioners, and other hair products, as well as oral finasteride, minoxidil solution and foam, ketoconazole shampoo, and other treatments for hair loss. Depending on the treatment selected, monthly costs start at $10. Find out more about Keeps.

Lemonaid: Lemonaid offers treatments for ED, PE, and hair loss in a manner that is comparable to that of Hims and Roman. Lemonaid ED medication costs $2, PE treatment costs $1, and hair loss treatments cost $60 for three months. Find out more regarding Lemonaid.

Questions about Hims and Roman that are frequently asked

Here are some frequently asked questions about telehealth companies, ED, and hair loss treatment.

Are there any other options for ED treatment?

According to the NIDDK-Trusted Source, ED may benefit from non-medicinal treatments. It suggests making some changes to one's lifestyle, like quitting smoking, drinking less alcohol, and staying active.

To help people get and keep an erection, other treatments, like vacuum erectile devices, may be considered. Every treatment option should be discussed with a doctor.

Is there anything else I can do to stop losing my hair?

Hair loss can be treated in a variety of ways, including:

Transplanting hair: A surgeon moves healthy hair from another area of the scalp to an area with thinning hair for this procedure.

Platelet-rich plasma: Plasma is injected into the scalp after being taken from the patient's blood and separated from the blood.

Laser gadgets: Laser devices that can be used at home to encourage hair growth are available from some businesses. Products that have been approved by the FDA should only be bought by people.

How safe are online pharmacies?

According to the FDA, a legitimate, safe pharmacy always has a physical address and phone number within the United States, requires a prescription from a licensed doctor, and is legal.

In addition, pharmacies should have a pharmacist who is licensed in the state where they do business and can answer questions from customers.

The FDA records online drug stores to avoid on its site.

Is Roman equivalent to Hims?

Roman and Hims are both telehealth organizations that offer internet based interviews with medical services experts who can endorse drugs for a few ailments.

However, Roman and Hims are owned and operated by various businesses. Individuals ought to consider which brand offers the medicine at the cost they see as generally OK prior to picking which organization to utilize.

Does Hims make you last longer?

Hims sells PE products like wipes and sprays for the climax delay. Before ejaculating, these products can help a person have more sex.

Roman or BlueChew, which is superior?

Telehealth providers Blue Chew and Roman both provide prescription ED medications.

Treatments for hair loss, mental health, skin care, a variety of sexual and primary care issues, and other issues are offered by Roman. Blue Chew, on the other hand, only offers the following ED medications: vardenafil, sildenafil, and tadalafil. All of these products are offered for sale in a chewable form, which is not approved by the FDA.

What can be done to make Hims last longer?

Two prescription medications for PE are available from Hims. These prescriptions are sertraline and paroxetine, which are a sort of upper called particular serotonin reuptake inhibitors (SSRIs). SSRIs can help prevent PE, according to research.

Hims and Roman are male-focused telehealth businesses that sell health products. Prescription ED medications, treatments for PE and hair loss, and nonprescription products for general health are some options.

In order to talk about prescriptions and any possible side effects, both businesses provide consultations and follow-up appointments with medical professionals. It is essential to report any side effects.

4 Safe Online Sources for Erectile Dysfunction (ED) Pills in 2023

The Food and Drug Administration (FDA) cautions against purchasing ED pills from websites that do not require a prescription. It is essential to select online retailers that require a prescription in order to steer clear of products containing harmful ingredients that are not listed.

As per the FDA, the quantity of ED items accessible on the web and in retail locations is expanding. Be that as it may, individuals ought to be careful and stay away from unregulated ED cures, including those makers guarantee to be "normal enhancements."

This article will see a few medications that assistance with ED, the dangers related with getting them on the web, and where to securely get ED pills. It will also talk about some other treatments for ED.

Best ED medications: What do they mean?

The majority of people can generally take erectile dysfunction (ED) pills that require a prescription from a local pharmacy safely. However, ED pills should be avoided by individuals who are taking nitrates to treat an existing heart condition.

PDE5 (phosphodiesterase) inhibitors can be found in ED pills. If these are taken with nitrates, a person may experience an unsafe drop in blood pressure.

PDE5 inhibitors assist an individual with accomplishing an erection by loosening up the smooth muscle in the walls of the veins. This enlargement permits the penis to load up with blood.

We discuss the various types of ED pills, their safety and side effects, and the distinctions between generic and brand-name options in this article.

Pills for erectile dysfunction

There are four main types of ED pills that have been approved as treatments in the United States by the Food and Drug Administration (FDA).

They are:

sildenafil (Viagra), tadalafil (Cialis), vardenafil (Levitra), and avanafil (Stendra) Viagra Sildenafil, more commonly referred to as Viagra, is frequently the initial treatment for erectile dysfunction (ED). Because it has been on the market for such a long time, Viagra's side effects and interactions are well-known, which is why doctors often prefer to try it before other treatments.

A lot of doctors recommend taking 50 milligrams (mg) of Viagra about an hour before having sex, according to Trusted Source. Be that as it may, it ought to be successful somewhere in the range of 30 minutes to 4 hours before sex.

Viagra's absorption rate will be slowed and its effects will be delayed if taken with food. Viagra should also not be taken with alcohol.

When a person takes Viagra, it typically takes between 30 and 120 minutes for it to start working.

Cialis

The underlying portion for Cilias is 10 mg, and an individual can accept it as essential for sexual movement. They can take as little as 5 milligrams or as much as 20 milligrams, depending on their requirements and tolerance.

Other ED medications behave differently than Cialis. Because it breaks down slower, it stays in the body longer.

BPH can be treated with Cialis at a dose of 5 milligrams from a doctor. As a result, it is an effective option for simultaneously treating ED and enlarged prostate symptoms.

A 2017 review by Trusted Source looked at 16 trials comparing Cialis and Viagra and found that people preferred taking Cialis because they felt less pressure to take it when they wanted to, which made them feel more confident in their sexuality.

Vardenafil is sold under the brand name Levitra. A first dose of 10 mg, taken one hour before sexual activity, is recommended by doctors. The greatest portion is 20 mg, with the base being 5 mg.

A specialist might change the portion contingent upon the drug's impact on the individual. An individual ought to take Levitra something like one time each day, regardless of food.

Vardenafil can be found in the tablet Staxyn, which dissolves. The FDA says that because it has a stronger effect on the body, it is "not interchangeable" with Levitra.

Staxyn comes in 10-mg tablets that disintegrate on the tongue. The tablet can be taken with or without food approximately one hour before sexual activity, but no more than one tablet should be taken per day.

Stendra

The following doses have been approved by the FDA: 50, 100, and 200 milligrams. Typically, a person takes Stendra 30 minutes before engaging in sexual activity. Depending on how well a person responds to treatment, the starting dose may be increased to 200 mg or decreased to 50 mg.

Are ED pills safe?

The clinical local area considers ED pills by and large safe for a great many people who are generally solid enough for sexual action.

A person may experience side effects, as is the case with any medication. Additionally, ED pills can interact with nitrates and other medications.

It is significant not to take ED pills with nitrates like dynamite, in light of the fact that the medications can communicate to cause hazardously low pulse.

Alpha-blockers and ED medications should be separated by four hours for people who suffer from urinary problems. Alpha-blockers incorporate doxazosin (Cardura) and prazosin (Minipress).

Do side effects exist?

There is a chance of mild side effects with each ED pill.

Some common side effects are:

Diarrhea, vision-related issues, flushing, nasal congestion, dizziness, headache, rash, upset stomach, and flushing are all signs of an erection that lasts longer than four hours. The penis may sustain permanent damage from an extended erection.

How effective are they?

70% of people taking ED medications, according to experts, will get an erection strong enough for sexual activity.

Other preexisting conditions, such as nerve damage from surgery or diabetes, will have an impact on the quality of the erection as well as the pleasure and sensations. However, those who are able to ejaculate should have an erection that lasts long enough for them.

How quickly do ED pills work?

Individuals will vary in how long it takes for ED pills to work. The majority of manufacturers advise patients to take their ED medication 15 to 60 minutes before engaging in sexual activity.

For the best erection, specialists suggest that an individual likewise participates in foreplay with their accomplice to assist with invigorating excitement.

Stendra, Viagra, Levitra, and Staxyn offer a more immediate sexual experience.

On the other hand, Cialis stays in the body for a longer period of time and takes longer to take full effect. Subsequently, great for individuals favor the unwavering quality of a day to day use item with longer-enduring impacts.

Options versus generics Brand-name medications are more well-known than generics because of advertising. They are typically more expensive than generic alternatives because they are first on the market. Because it takes time to release their patent rights, generic versions of newer medications typically do not exist.

Generics are imitations of brand-name products. The effects and dosage instructions of a generic medication are identical to those of a brand-name medication. In order to save money, an individual's insurance company may substitute a generic version for the brand-name counterpart.

A reputable pharmacy should always be used to buy medications. Prescriptions are required to purchase

ED medications. People shouldn't buy them if they are available online without a prescription.

Pills for erectile dysfunction that are being sold illegally may originate from an untrustworthy manufacturing facility and may contain a potentially hazardous mix of ingredients.

Frequently Asked Questions about ED Pills

In this section, we address some frequently Asked Questions regarding these medications.

Which medication for erectile dysfunction has the fewest adverse effects?

Every drug for ED can have side effects.

However, sildenafil is typically prescribed by doctors first.

What is the main erectile brokenness pill?

A medical care proficient will help an individual chooses the best erectile brokenness pill for their conditions.

Cost, side effects, formulation, how frequently a person needs to take the medication, and whether a person is happy using generic or brand-name medications are all factors to consider when selecting the best erectile dysfunction pill.

What is the best treatment for elderly ED?

According to Research, modifying one's lifestyle factors, such as quitting smoking, losing weight if necessary, and exercising regularly, is the first step in treating ED in seniors.

PDE5 inhibitors, such as sildenafil and tadalafil, are frequently used to alleviate the symptoms of erectile dysfunction (ED) in older people. Seniors shouldn't take this kind of medication unless they also take nitrates or have a high risk of cardiovascular disease that makes it hard to exercise.

How can I regain my ability to erect?

There are a few techniques an individual might use to have and keep an erection.

Reduced symptoms of erectile dysfunction (ED) may be aided by making changes to one's lifestyle, such as exercising regularly, following a healthy diet, avoiding alcohol, and controlling conditions like diabetes and high blood pressure.

Penis pumps may help maintain erections for some people. A recent report viewed that as 77% of individuals and their accomplices were happy with the result in the wake of utilizing these gadgets.

However, before using any of these devices, individuals should always consult with a medical professional.

In a nutshell, medications for erectile dysfunction generally don't cause any serious side effects. Most of the time, the drugs work the same way and help people get an erection for sexual activity.

Individuals ought to survey every one of their drugs with a specialist and examine safe choices in the event that they are taking alpha-blockers or nitrates. This is critical because taking these medications together could result in a dangerous drop in blood pressure.

Viagra, Cialis, Levitra, and Stendra: Which is better?

For the treatment of erectile dysfunction (ED) symptoms, four well-known medications are widely available.

The medications are phosphodiesterase 5 (PDE5) inhibitors, and the brand names for them are Viagra (sildenafil), Cialis (tadalafil), Levitra (vardenafil), and Stendra (avanafil). The generic names for the drugs are Stendra (avanafil).

They all serve the same purpose and have received approval from the Food and Drug Administration (FDA). Nevertheless, they differ in a few ways.

Understanding these distinctions can assist an individual with picking the most reasonable choice.

How do drugs for ED work?

All of the drugs work in a similar way because they are PDE5 inhibitors. They assist with loosening up the muscles and increment blood stream to the body.

People with ED are able to have a long-lasting erection during sexual activity because this makes it easier for blood to enter the penis.

The drugs work quickly, but the exact timing varies from drug to drug.

This table shows when to take the medication, the standard beginning portion in milligrams (mg), and how lengthy the impact is probably going to endure. It should be noted that a doctor may alter the dose for individuals taking other medications and those with particular health conditions.

Cialis and Lemonaid Health Lemonaid Health provides a variety of ED medications, including daily Cialis and generic versions of Viagra and Cialis.

A person must respond to an online survey in order to use this service. Before developing a treatment plan, the medical team reviews the patient's medical history and may inquire further.

According to Lemonaid Health, its ED medications start at $2 per pill. For people who have sex more than five times per week, the company suggests taking generic daily Cialis.

The organization offers free conveyance. Lemonaid Health informs customers that if they select delivery, they will be required to pay for their prescriptions out of their own pockets. A person can request that the prescription be sent to a nearby pharmacy instead if the medication is covered by their health insurance.

Viagra and the Optum Store Viagra, Cialis, Levitra, and Stendra: Which is better?

Side effects Drug interactions Changes in lifestyle

Getting in touch with a doctor FAQ Summary We include products that we believe our readers will find useful. We may receive a small commission if you make a purchase through the links on this page. Here is our procedure.

How we vet brands and items

Four well known drugs are generally accessible for treating the side effects of erectile brokenness (ED).

The medications are phosphodiesterase 5 (PDE5) inhibitors, and the brand names for them are Viagra (sildenafil), Cialis (tadalafil), Levitra (vardenafil), and

Stendra (avanafil). The generic names for the drugs are Stendra (avanafil).

They all serve the same purpose and have received approval from the Food and Drug Administration (FDA). Nevertheless, they differ in a few ways.

Understanding these distinctions can assist an individual with picking the most reasonable choice.

In our dedicated hub, learn more about ED and premature ejaculation.

How do drugs for ED work?

All of the drugs work in a similar way because they are PDE5 inhibitors. They assist with loosening up the muscles and increment blood stream to the body.

People with ED are able to have a long-lasting erection during sexual activity because this makes it easier for blood to enter the penis

The drugs work quickly, but the exact timing varies from drug to drug.

This table shows when to take the medication, the standard beginning portion in milligrams (mg), and how lengthy the impact is probably going to endure. It should be noted that a doctor may alter the dose for individuals taking other medications and those with particular health conditions.

Cialis versus Viagra

The accompanying table analyzes these two ED meds:

Tadalafil sildenafil is the main ingredient in Cialis and Viagra. It takes about 30 minutes for it to work (trusted source); it lasts about 4 to 12 hours (trusted source); it can be taken daily, at the same time each day; it can be taken with or without food; it lasts longer than Viagra; it can be taken daily; it only needs to be taken when you want to have sex (trusted source); sildenafil is one of the There are two choices that people might think about:

Cialis and Lemonaid Health

Lemonaid Health provides a variety of ED medications, including daily Cialis and generic versions of Viagra and Cialis.

A person must respond to an online survey in order to use this service. Before developing a treatment plan, the medical team reviews the patient's medical history and may inquire further.

According to Lemonaid Health, its ED medications start at $2 per pill. For people who have sex more than five times per week, the company suggests taking generic daily Cialis.

The organization offers free conveyance. Lemonaid Health informs customers that if they select delivery, they will be required to pay for their prescriptions out of their own pockets. A person can request that the prescription be sent to a nearby pharmacy instead if the medication is covered by their health insurance.

Optum Store and Viagra

We incorporate items we believe are helpful for our perusers. On the off chance that you purchase through joins on this page, we might procure a little commission or other unmistakable advantage. RVO Health owns Optum Store, Optum Perks, and Healthline Media. Our method is as follows:

Viagra and sildenafil, among other ED medications, are available at Optum Store.

Individuals should have a legitimate remedy to get ED prescriptions. The individuals who don't can select to finish up a web-based evaluation at Optum Store, which is then inspected by a medical services proficient. For people who qualify, an ED drug is endorsed and sent through mail. Additionally, if you have any inquiries, you can reach a pharmacist at any time.

The price of 30 20-mg tablets of sildenafil, also known as generic Viagra, at the company starts at $16. The cost of 30 25 mg Viagra tablets starts at $2,874.

At this time, only United Healthcare insurance plans are accepted by Optum Store.

The organization offers transporting for a level expense of $5.99, or $9.99 for sped up conveyance. On orders over $75, shipping is free.

Levitra vs. Viagra

These medications can also be purchased online from reputable telehealth providers with a valid prescription.

Levitra and Blink Health

Blink Health says it can help people find cheaper prescriptions and offers telemedicine appointments.

The business asserts that its ED medication prices are up to 50% lower than those of other health websites.

The first visit to the doctor and the first month of medication cost $10, and monthly refills cost $17.

It states that generic Viagra and Cialis are the most frequently prescribed medications by healthcare professionals on this platform.

Flicker Wellbeing states that vardenafil, the conventional type of Levitra, begins at $622.12 for 30 tablets of 20 mg.

Hims and Viagra Hims is a company that focuses on male health through telehealth. Viagra is one of the ED medications offered by the platform.

Hims sells branded Viagra for $139 per pill and generic Viagra for $3 per pill.

To begin with Hims, individuals must complete an online survey. People will be able to get in touch with a licensed doctor, who can give them treatment if it's necessary.

The organization offers free and prudent conveyance.

Stendra versus Viagra

Both Stendra and Viagra are available from the following telehealth providers:

Flicker Wellbeing and Stendra

Flicker Wellbeing states that it can assist with peopling track down the most minimal cost for their ED prescription.

The service does not specify whether Stendra is prescribed as part of its ED treatment plan, despite the fact that it offers ED treatment directly from the website for as little as $17 per month.

Instead, Stendra prescriptions can be sent to participating local pharmacies by Blink Health.

Through this platform, a bottle containing six 200 mg Stendra tablets costs $414.33.

Roman and Viagra

Roman provides generic Cialis and Viagra.

An online questionnaire must be completed before treatment can begin with this company. Roman will connect individuals with a medical professional who will, if necessary, prescribe treatment.

Conventional Viagra is accessible beginning from $4 per portion.

Rooman offers free and watchful two-day transporting.

Cost of ED medications

The medications used to treat ED can cost a lot of different things, depending on which one is chosen and whether the generic or brand-name version is used.

Costs will likewise differ contingent upon whether an individual's protection wil cover the cost of the prescription. Individuals ought to continuously contact their protection supplier to see which drug it covers. A few organizations may not offer inclusion for marked medicine.

Sites, for example, Optum Advantages find and analyze costs of prescription and may offer limits and coupons. Individuals might find their drug at a less expensive cost utilizing an examination site.

Who are ED drugs for?

The drugs Stendra, Viagra, Cialis, and Levitra are all used to treat ED symptoms.

If a person meets one of the following criteria, a doctor will diagnose ED:

Always being unable to get an erection

Frequently being not able to get an erection

Having the option to get an erection yet one that doesn't keep going long enough for sex

Parts of physical and psychological wellness can add to ED, and a specialist will examine these and way of life propensities with the person prior to endorsing these medications.

If a person has a cardiovascular condition that makes sexual activity dangerous, doctors may not prescribe the drugs.

Additionally, they should not be combined with other medications. Find out more about the medications that may interact with these ones below.

Comparing side effects, Viagra, Cialis, Levitra, and Stendra all have many side effects and interactions that are similar to one another, but there are also some differences.

Anybody considering utilizing these medications ought to talk with a specialist first. Because they may interact with other medications or affect existing health conditions, the drugs may not be appropriate for everyone.

A person who has been told not to have sex because of cardiovascular problems or because they are taking nitrates for a heart condition is not a good candidate for any of these medications.

Combining these medications with nitrates or alpha-blockers may cause a sudden drop in blood pressure, which can cause fainting, dizziness, and even falls and injuries.

According to a previous study on rodents, the following medications may increase the body's concentration of PDE5 inhibitors. As a result, individuals who use ED drugs with any of these medications should consult a doctor first:

Ketoconazole, an antifungal and anti-dandruff agent, HIV protease inhibitors like ritonavir, and the antibiotics erythromycin and clarithromycin. Grapefruit juice is a CYP3A4 inhibitor, so it may enhance the effects of these medications.

In the event that an individual encounters vision misfortune, priapism, or unexpected hearing misfortune while utilizing any of these prescriptions, it is critical to contact crisis administrations for sure fire clinical consideration.

Comparing drug interactions

Each of the medications in this article has the potential to cause adverse interactions with other medications. To reduce the likelihood of adverse drug interactions, it is essential to inform a healthcare professional of any other medications a person is taking.

Viagra drug connections

Viagra might associate with the accompanying medications:

Alpha-blockers, such as nitroglycerin, medications to lower blood pressure; CYP4 inhibitors, such as ritonavir, ketoconazole, and erythromycin; nitrates, such as nitroglycerin; Cialis interactions and warnings

CYP3A4 inducers, such as rifampin, an antibiotic, as they may prevent Cialis from working CYP3A4 inhibitors, such as ketoconazole and ritonavir, as they can increase the impact Levitra interactions and warnings Individuals should not use Levitra if they have an irregular heartbeat or are using the following:

Drugs to lower blood pressure that contain nitrates and alpha-blockers. If a person has liver problems or is already taking one of the following drugs:

Antifungal medications like ketoconazole or itraconazole, antibiotics like clarithromycin or erythromycin, and antiretroviral medications like ritonavir, indinavir, saquinavir, or atazanavir, which doctors use to treat or prevent HIV Stendra interactions and warnings: A person should not take Stendra with nitrates or any strong CYP3A4 inhibitors like ketoconazole or riton

A specialist might change the portion in the event that an individual is utilizing alpha-blockers or a moderate CYP3A4 inhibitor, like erythromycin, amprenavir, or diltiazem.

Because they can cause a drop in blood pressure, the following should be avoided when taking Stendra:

Alpha-blockers for high blood pressure alcohol other concerns Individuals should also ensure that their product is an approved version and follow a doctor's instructions when purchasing any of these medications.

In 2020, for instance, the FDA exhorted individuals not to buy an imported item sold as an enhancement called U.S.A Viagra.

The Food and Drug Administration (FDA) issued a warning about this product, noting that while it contains sildenafil, it is not a form of Viagra that has been approved. As a result, it may pose a risk, particularly to individuals who suffer from certain health conditions or who are taking medications that

Changes in lifestyle

While these medications can assist in the management of erectile dysfunction (ED), a doctor may advise attempting to modify one's lifestyle first.

Trusted Source is one strategy that has the potential to improve ED.

reaching or maintaining a moderate body weight avoiding the use of some recreational drugs seeking counseling to help manage anxiety and stress When to contact a doctor It is advisable, according to Trusted Source, for anyone who has concerns about ED to consult a doctor because they may be able to assist. Limiting alcohol consumption, if applicable. One of these drugs, for instance, may be prescribed by them.

If a person is already taking one of these medications, they should see a doctor if the medication doesn't work or if they have side effects like changing their vision. The dosage or type of medication may need to be altered by the doctor.

People ought to look for sure fire clinical consideration on the off chance that they experience any of the accompanying:

Viagra, Cialis, Levitra, and Stendra can help a person get an erection, but they will not cure ED. Other medications include priapism, hearing loss, vision loss, and priapism. Therapy with testosterone and, in some instances, surgery, two additional potential treatments.

As often as possible posed inquiries about Cialis and Viagra

Beneath, we respond to probably the most widely recognized inquiries regarding Viagra, Cialis, Levitra, and Stendra.

Which is superior? Levitra, Viagra, Cialis, or Stendra?

The decision will be based on the individual as well as a number of factors, such as whether or not the individual has sex on a regular basis, any other medications they are taking, and the price and availability of ED medications.

A healthcare professional should be consulted by individuals before making a decision.

Do these medications make you greater?

They don't really. During an erection, they increase blood flow to the penis but do not alter its size.

Which pill is more effective?

Cialis (tadalafil) has effects that last up to 36 hours, but this only means that a person can have one or more erections during that time. It does not imply that they will experience a 36-hour erection.

Is Cialis more compelling than Viagra?

Studies show that both Cialis and Viagra's active ingredients, tadalafil and sildenafil, boost a person's sexual confidence. Both drugs have similar efficacy profiles.

However, the longer-lasting effects of tadalafil make it a preferred choice for both the drug's users and their partners.

Is Cialis more potent than Viagra?

Although Cialis has a longer mechanism of action than Viagra, it will not assist users in achieving stronger erections.

How long does Cialis take to reach its peak effect?

The producers of Cialis suggest taking the prescription something like 30 minutes before sexual movement.

Is 100 mg of Viagra equivalent to 20 mg of Cialis?

The maximum dosage for Cialis is 20 milligrams. The maximum dosage that can be prescribed by a medical professional is 100 mg of Viagra.

Without consulting a medical professional, patients should never switch medications.

Viagra, Levitra, Cialis, and Stendra can assist an individual with ED get and keep an erection.

There are numerous interactions and side effects to take into account. On the other hand, these drugs can help a person get over ED and have sex.

It should be noted that none of these drugs will stimulate sexual desire. To get an erection, the person will need stimulation.

Trial and error may be the only method for selecting the best drug. Working straightforwardly with a specialist can assist an individual with following secondary effects and conclude which medication is generally reasonable for them.

Erectile Dysfunction Treatment

Is there a way to treat erectile dysfunction?

You can treat an underlying cause of your erectile dysfunction (ED) with the help of a medical professional. The choice of ED treatment is up to the individual. In any case, you likewise may profit from talking with your accomplice about which treatment is best for you as a team.

Changes to your lifestyle

Your healthcare provider may recommend that you make changes to your lifestyle to help reduce or improve ED. You can limit or stop drinking alcohol, quit smoking, increase physical activity, maintain a healthy weight, and stop using illegal drugs. If you have trouble making these changes on your own, you can get help from a health professional.

Go to guiding

Consult with your primary care physician about going to a guide in the event that mental or intense subject matters are influencing your ED. A guide can show you how to bring down your nervousness NIH outer connection or stress connected with sex. You may be advised by your counselor to bring your partner to counseling sessions so that they can learn how to support you. As you work on easing your nervousness or stress, a specialist can zero in on treating the actual reasons for ED.

How is erectile dysfunction treated by doctors?

Change your medications If ED is caused by a medication you take for another condition, your doctor may recommend a different dose or another medication. Take constantly a medication without talking with your PCP first. Find out about which drugs cause it almost certain that you'll to foster ED.

Prescribe oral medications

A doctor might give you a prescription for an oral medication, also known as a medication taken orally, like one of the following to help you get and keep an erection:

Prescribe medicines and suppositories that can be injected. Many men find that by injecting a drug called alprostadil NIH external link into their penis, which makes it full of blood, they get stronger erections. Although oral medications may enhance your response to sexual stimulation, unlike injectable medications, they do not automatically produce an erection.

Some men insert an alprostadil suppository into the urethra rather than injecting a drug. A suppository is a solid medication that is injected into the body, where it dissolves. You will be given a prefilled applicator by a medical professional so that you can insert the pellet about an inch into your urethra. An erection will start inside 8 to 10 minutes and may last 30 to an hour.

Talk about alternative medicines

Some men say that taking certain alternative medicines orally can help them get and keep an erection. However, not all "natural" supplements and medications are secure. Blends of specific endorsed and elective meds could cause significant medical issues. Talk to a health care professional about your use of alternative medicines, such as vitamin and mineral supplements, to help ensure safe and coordinated care. Additionally, consult your physician before placing an online medication order.

How will I be affected by medications for erectile dysfunction side effects?

Side effects of ED medications that are taken orally, via injection, or as a pellet in the urethra can include priapism, a persistent erection. Call a medical services proficient immediately in the event that an erection endures 4 hours or longer.

After taking oral ED medications, a small percentage of men experience vision or hearing impairment. Call your medical care proficient immediately assuming you foster these issues.

www.ingramcontent.com/pod-product-compliance
Lightning Source LLC
Chambersburg PA
CBHW070452220526
45466CB00004B/1804